MY ROUTE TO HEALTH SECTIONS

📅	**4 WEEK PLAN / CALENDAR**	**PAGE 4**
🏋	**GOALS**	**PAGE 5**
📝	**MY JOURNAL**	**PAGE 7**
🍎	**HEALTHY EATING**	**PAGE 17**
🚴	**EXERCISE PLAN**	**PAGE 33**

WELCOME!

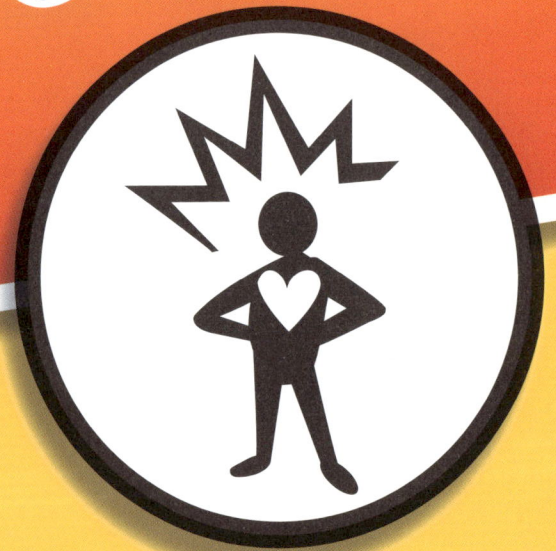

You have stepped in the right direction to get on track with your overall health. Your "Route to Health" will provide direction and tools to help with goal setting, tracking your progress on a calendar for four weeks, encouraging tips to get active, redirecting your focus on your health and giving you a road map for daily healthy habits. Making small changes in your life can go a long way. Remember, this book is just a guideline to help you get started on your "Route to Health," but make sure to use it in a way that will help you stay on course with your goals. Always talk to your doctor before starting any exercise or activity program, or before making changes to your diet. Listen to your doctor's advice regarding exercise and nutrition. Your doctor can consider any health conditions while you take your "Route to Health."

THE FOOD PYRAMID

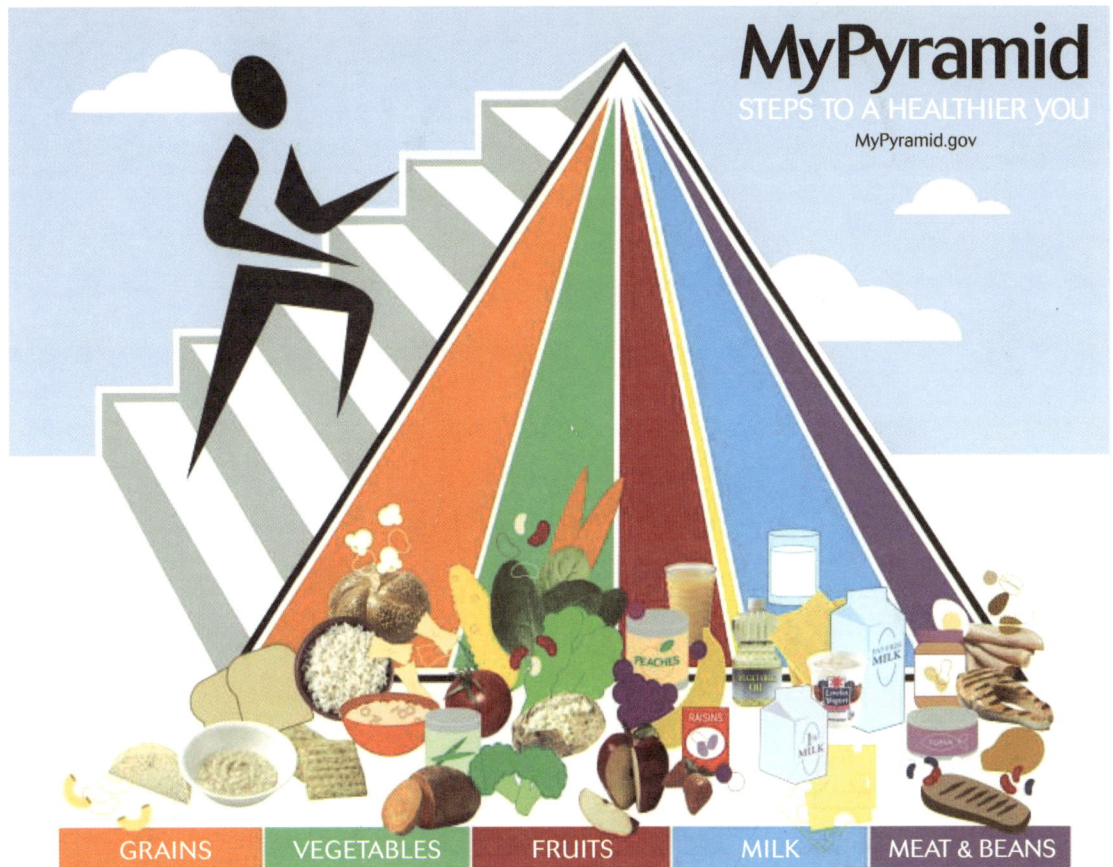

MyPyramid
STEPS TO A HEALTHIER YOU
MyPyramid.gov

GRAINS	VEGETABLES	FRUITS	MILK	MEAT & BEANS

GRAINS	VEGETABLES	FRUITS	MILK	MEAT & BEANS
Make half your grains whole	Vary your veggies	Focus on fruits	Get your calcium-rich foods	Go lean with protein
Eat at least 3 oz. of whole-grain cereals, breads, crackers, rice, or pasta every day 1 oz. is about 1 slice of bread, about 1 cup of breakfast cereal, or ½ cup of cooked rice, cereal, or pasta	Eat more dark-green veggies like broccoli, spinach, and other dark leafy greens Eat more orange vegetables like carrots and sweetpotatoes Eat more dry beans and peas like pinto beans, kidney beans, and lentils	Eat a variety of fruit Choose fresh, frozen, canned, or dried fruit Go easy on fruit juices	Go low-fat or fat-free when you choose milk, yogurt, and other milk products If you don't or can't consume milk, choose lactose-free products or other calcium sources such as fortified foods and beverages	Choose low-fat or lean meats and poultry Bake it, broil it, or grill it Vary your protein routine — choose more fish, beans, peas, nuts, and seeds

For a 2,000-calorie diet, you need the amounts below from each food group. To find the amounts that are right for you, go to MyPyramid.gov.

Eat 6 oz. every day	Eat 2½ cups every day	Eat 2 cups every day	Get 3 cups every day; for kids aged 2 to 8, it's 2	Eat 5½ oz. every day

Find your balance between food and physical activity
- Be sure to stay within your daily calorie needs.
- Be physically active for at least 30 minutes most days of the week.
- About 60 minutes a day of physical activity may be needed to prevent weight gain.
- For sustaining weight loss, at least 60 to 90 minutes a day of physical activity may be required.
- Children and teenagers should be physically active for 60 minutes every day, or most days.

Know the limits on fats, sugars, and salt (sodium)
- Make most of your fat sources from fish, nuts, and vegetable oils.
- Limit solid fats like butter, margarine, shortening, and lard, as well as foods that contain them.
- Check the Nutrition Facts label to keep saturated fats, trans fats, and sodium low.
- Choose food and beverages low in added sugars. Added sugars contribute calories with few, if any, nutrients.

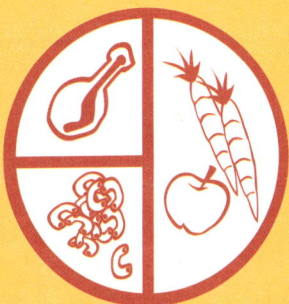

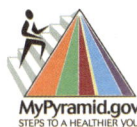

MyPyramid.gov
STEPS TO A HEALTHIER YOU

U.S. Department of Agriculture
Center for Nutrition Policy and Promotion
April 2005
CNPP-15

USDA

HEALTHY EATING CONSISTS OF A BALANCED DIET.
HERE ARE SOME HEALTHY EXAMPLES FROM EACH FOOD GROUP:

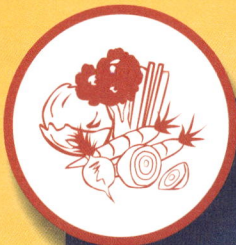

Vegetables

FOOD FOR THOUGHT: Make sure to eat more fresh vegetables that are dark green!

BROCCOLI, SPINACH, DARK LEAFY GREENS. CARROTS, SWEET POTATOES, BEANS, PEAS

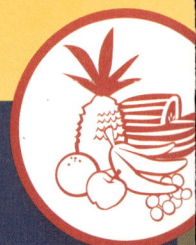

Fruits

FOOD FOR THOUGHT: Eat a wide variety of fruits that are fresh, frozen or canned-with light syrup!

GRAPES, BANANAS, PEACHES, STRAWBERRIES, APPLES, ORANGES. WATERMELONS

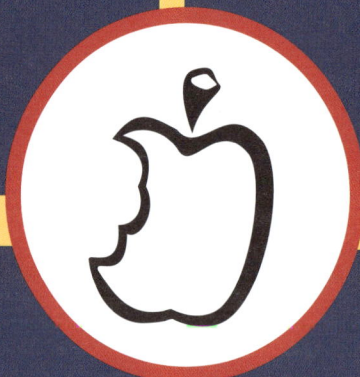

Milk/Dairy

FOOD FOR THOUGHT: It is best to choose fat free or low fat items most of the time!

LOW FAT MILK, 2% MILK, LOW FAT MOZZARELLA CHEESE, LOW FAT YOGURT

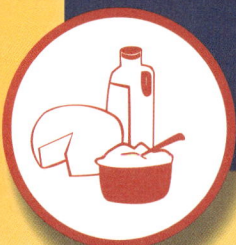

Grains

FOOD FOR THOUGHT: When choosing grains, it's better to eat multigrain or wheat instead of white bread or foods made from white flour.

WHOLE WHEAT TORTILLAS, WHOLE WHEAT BREAD, MULTIGRAIN CEREAL, BROWN RICE, ENRICHED PASTA, FULLY COOKED OATMEAL

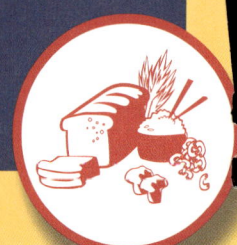

SOME FOOD CHOICES ARE BETTER THAN OTHERS ON YOUR ROUTE TO HEALTH

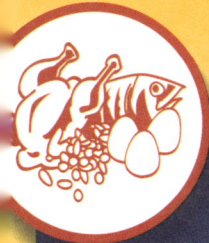

Meats, Eggs, Beans

FOOD FOR THOUGHT: When you eat meat as a protein source it is important to choose a lean version.

CHICKEN, FISH, TURKEY, LEAN HAM, BOILED EGGS, BEANS, NUTS, LEAN BEEF

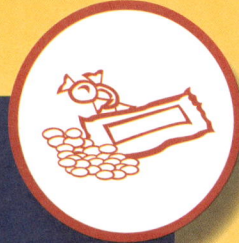

Liquids

FOOD FOR THOUGHT: Liquids are essential for your body, but make sure they are fueling it with nutrition and not filling it with empty calories

FAT-FREE MILK, 1% LOW-FAT MILK, WATER, DIET SODA, UNSWEETENED ICE TEA, DIET ICE TEA, SUGAR FREE LEMONADE

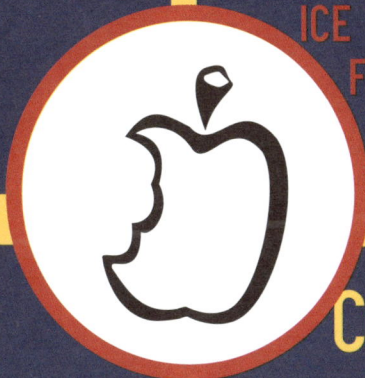

Fats & Oils

FOOD FOR THOUGHT: Everyone needs a small amount of fat or oil in their diet. Healthier oils come from fish or nuts.

VEGETABLE OIL, CORN OIL, LOW-FAT MARGARINE, OLIVE OIL

Condiments & Sauces

FOOD FOR THOUGHT: Instead of using fatty condiments or sauces, try adding zest to your meal with spices.

KETCHUP, SALSA, MUSTARD, FAT-FREE SALAD DRESSING, FAT-FREE MAYONNAISE, FAT-FREE SOUR CREAM, LIGHT SOY SAUCE, WORCESTERSHIRE SAUCE

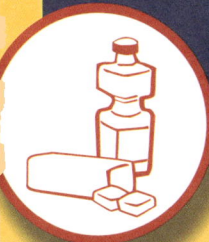

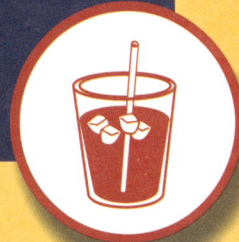

"Divide & Conquer Your Plate!"

WHAT IS HEALTHY PART OF YOUR

MEATS, EGGS, BEANS & FISH
5 1/2 OUNCES DAILY

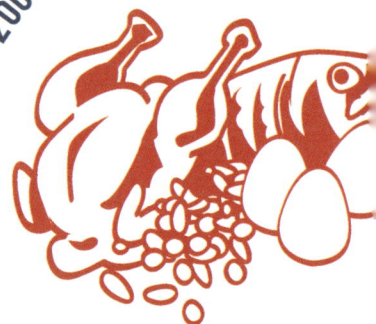

Egg whites, egg substitutes are the best choice. Omelettes, boiled or poached eggs.

Kidney beans, split peas, red beans, navy beans, lentils and tofu.

Chicken and turkey without the skin- broiled, baked or grilled.

Tuna canned in water. Baked, broiled, steamed or grilled fish and shellfish.

Chicken and turkey without the skin-broiled, baked or grilled.

Trimmed and lean beef and pork.

For meat, 3 ounces is about the size of a deck of playing cards.

1 ounce is the same as 1 egg or 1 tablespoon of peanut butter.

GRAINS
6 OUNCES DAILY

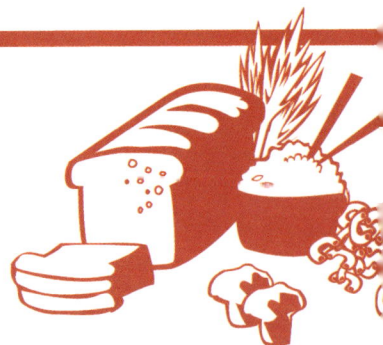

Whole wheat and multigrain are your best choice instead of white bread.

Whole wheat or multigrain sandwich bread, english muffins, crackers, tortillas, pasta or buns.

Steel cut oatmeal and brown rice are your best options.

In your recipes that call for white flour, try substituting whole wheat flour.

1 ounce equals about 1 slice of bread, 1 cup of breakfast cereal, or 1/2 cup of cooked rice, cereal or pasta.

WEBSITES FOR MORE HEALTHY EATING INFO:
www.startsmartforyourhealth.com
www.mypyramid.gov

AT FROM EACH
DED PLATE?

FRUITS
2 CUPS DAILY

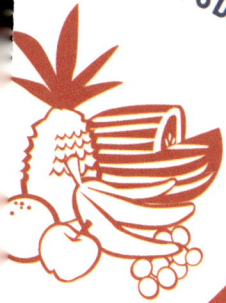

VEGETABLES
2 1/2 CUPS DAILY

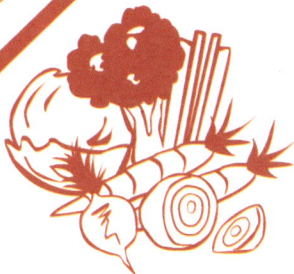

MILK/DAIRY
3 CUPS DAILY

FATS & OILS
LIMITED DAILY INTAKE

Fresh fruit, frozen or canned in natural juice with no sugar.

Fruit salad topped with low fat yogurt.

Sliced apples and low fat peanut butter.

Raisins, prunes, figs and dates.

Baked, steamed, raw broiled or boiled green beans, peas, celery, broccoli, asparagus, spinach, brussels sprouts, cauliflower, zucchini and carrots.

Baked, boiled, grilled potatoes and sweet potatoes.

Fresh, frozen and canned vegetables steamed or boiled without added sauces, fat, oils or butter.

Spinach, romaine or bib lettuce make a great salad if you add carrots, onions, cucumber, tomatoes, mushrooms, green/yellow/red peppers and celery.

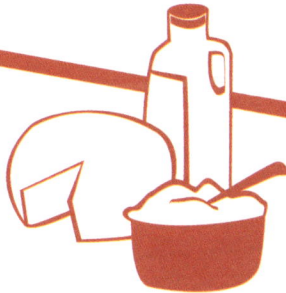

1.5 ounces of cheese is the same thing as 1 cup of milk.

Fat free or low fat milk, yogurt or cottage cheese or half and half.

Cooking with small amounts of vegetable oil is better than using butter or shortening.

Fats that come from fish, nuts or vegetable oils are the best choice.

Q: WHAT ABOUT WATER?

A: IT'S ALL ABOUT WATER!

Just the facts...about H_2O!

* Water flushes out the bad stuff in your body called toxins
* Water helps carry nutrients from food and vitamins to your body's cells
* Water helps the moisture and health of your ears, nose, throat and skin

THREE GOOD RULES ABOUT WATER:

1) Remember "8 x 8." Eight ounces of water, eight times a day. Sounds like a lot, but here's an easy way to tackle the 8 x 8: Drink a glass of water... when you wake up... mid morning... with lunch (2 glasses)... afternoon... dinner (2 glasses)... mid evening/before bedtime.

2) Drink enough so you rarely feel thirsty

3) If you exercise, it's important to put the water you sweat out back into your body. Make sure to drink before, during and after exercise to stay hydrated!

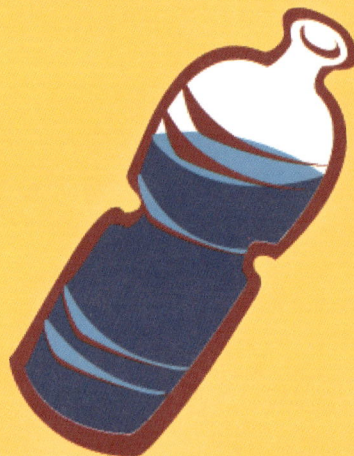

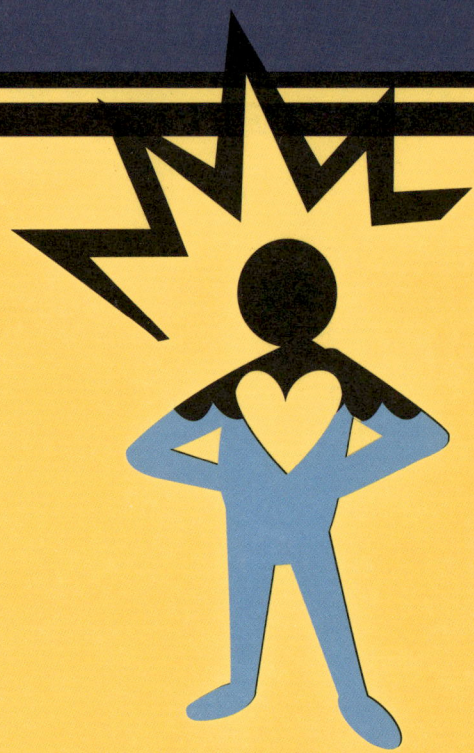

YOUR BODY IS 60% WATER!

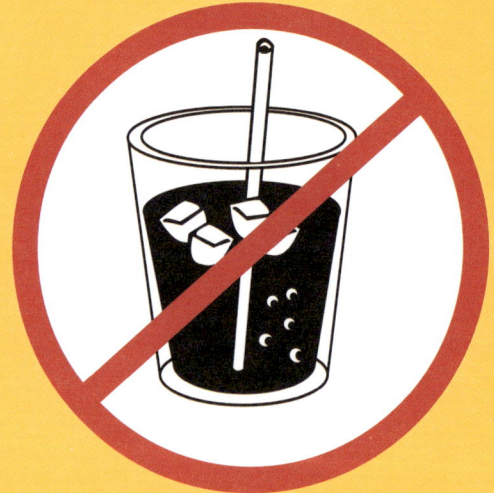

NOT SO HEALTHY LIQUIDS...

GO with H_2O over these choices:

Sweetened ice tea
Fruit punch
Powdered sugary drink mixes
Sugary sodas

SHOPPING LIST WEEK 1

MILK & DAIRY

- [ ] fat free or low fat milk
- [ ] low fat yogurt
- [ ] low fat cheese
- [ ] cottage cheese
- [ ] margarine

BREADS & GRAINS

- [ ] whole wheat bread
- [ ] whole wheat english muffins
- [ ] corn tortillas
- [ ] whole wheat tortillas
- [ ] multigrain cereal
- [ ] brown rice
- [ ] enriched pasta

MEATS & BEANS

- [ ] white meat chicken (no skin)
- [ ] white meat turkey
- [ ] lean beef
- [ ] pinto beans
- [ ] navy beans
- [ ] black beans
- [ ] fish
- [ ] eggs

FRUITS

- [ ] bananas
- [ ] grapes
- [ ] oranges
- [ ] pears
- [ ] peaches
- [ ] strawberries
- [ ] apples
- [ ] canned fruit in light syrup
- [ ] watermelon
- [ ] cherries

VEGETABLES

- [ ] carrots
- [ ] broccoli
- [ ] spinach
- [ ] lettuce
- [ ] tomatoes
- [ ] green beans
- [ ] collard greens
- [ ] celery
- [ ] peppers
- [ ] onions
- [ ] mushrooms
- [ ] cucumbers
- [ ] canned or frozen vegetables (no salt)

FATS, OILS & SAUCES

- [ ] salsa
- [ ] low or non fat salad dressing
- [ ] mustard
- [ ] vegetable oil
- [ ] vinegar

WEEK 1
OTHER ITEMS

OTHER ITEMS

MILK & DAIRY

- [ ] fat free or low fat milk
- [ ] low fat yogurt
- [ ] low fat cheese
- [ ] cottage cheese
- [ ] margarine

BREADS & GRAINS

- [ ] whole wheat bread
- [ ] whole wheat english muffins
- [ ] corn tortillas
- [ ] whole wheat tortillas
- [ ] multigrain cereal
- [ ] brown rice
- [ ] enriched pasta

MEATS & BEANS

- [ ] white meat chicken (no skin)
- [ ] white meat turkey
- [ ] lean beef
- [ ] pinto beans
- [ ] navy beans
- [ ] black beans
- [ ] fish
- [ ] eggs

FRUITS

- [ ] bananas
- [ ] grapes
- [ ] oranges
- [ ] pears
- [ ] peaches
- [ ] strawberries
- [ ] apples
- [ ] canned fruit in light syrup
- [ ] watermelon
- [ ] cherries

VEGETABLES

- [ ] carrots
- [ ] broccoli
- [ ] spinach
- [ ] lettuce
- [ ] tomatoes
- [ ] green beans
- [ ] collard greens
- [ ] celery
- [ ] peppers
- [ ] onions
- [ ] mushrooms
- [ ] cucumbers
- [ ] canned or frozen vegetables (no salt)

FATS, OILS & SAUCES

- [ ] salsa
- [ ] low or non fat salad dressing
- [ ] mustard
- [ ] vegetable oil
- [ ] vinegar

WEEK 2
OTHER ITEMS

OTHER ITEMS

MILK & DAIRY

- ☐ fat free or low fat milk
- ☐ low fat yogurt
- ☐ low fat cheese
- ☐ cottage cheese
- ☐ margarine

BREADS & GRAINS

- ☐ whole wheat bread
- ☐ whole wheat english muffins
- ☐ corn tortillas
- ☐ whole wheat tortillas
- ☐ multigrain cereal
- ☐ brown rice
- ☐ enriched pasta

MEATS & BEANS

- ☐ white meat chicken (no skin)
- ☐ white meat turkey
- ☐ lean beef
- ☐ pinto beans
- ☐ navy beans
- ☐ black beans
- ☐ fish
- ☐ eggs

FRUITS

- ☐ bananas
- ☐ grapes
- ☐ oranges
- ☐ pears
- ☐ peaches
- ☐ strawberries
- ☐ apples
- ☐ canned fruit in light syrup
- ☐ watermelon
- ☐ cherries

VEGETABLES

- ☐ carrots
- ☐ broccoli
- ☐ spinach
- ☐ lettuce
- ☐ tomatoes
- ☐ green beans
- ☐ collard greens
- ☐ celery
- ☐ peppers
- ☐ onions
- ☐ mushrooms
- ☐ cucumbers
- ☐ canned or frozen vegetables (no salt)

FATS, OILS & SAUCES

- ☐ salsa
- ☐ low or non fat salad dressing
- ☐ mustard
- ☐ vegetable oil
- ☐ vinegar

WEEK 3
OTHER ITEMS

OTHER ITEMS

MILK & DAIRY

- [ ] fat free or low fat milk
- [ ] low fat yogurt
- [ ] low fat cheese
- [ ] cottage cheese
- [ ] margarine

BREADS & GRAINS

- [ ] whole wheat bread
- [ ] whole wheat english muffins
- [ ] corn tortillas
- [ ] whole wheat tortillas
- [ ] multigrain cereal
- [ ] brown rice
- [ ] enriched pasta

MEATS & BEANS

- [ ] white meat chicken (no skin)
- [ ] white meat turkey
- [ ] lean beef
- [ ] pinto beans
- [ ] navy beans
- [ ] black beans
- [ ] fish
- [ ] eggs

FRUITS

- [ ] bananas
- [ ] grapes
- [ ] oranges
- [ ] pears
- [ ] peaches
- [ ] strawberries
- [ ] apples
- [ ] canned fruit in light syrup
- [ ] watermelon
- [ ] cherries

VEGETABLES

- [ ] carrots
- [ ] broccoli
- [ ] spinach
- [ ] lettuce
- [ ] tomatoes
- [ ] green beans
- [ ] canned or frozen vegetables (no salt)
- [ ] collard greens
- [ ] celery
- [ ] peppers
- [ ] onions
- [ ] mushrooms
- [ ] cucumbers

FATS, OILS & SAUCES

- [ ] salsa
- [ ] low or non fat salad dressing
- [ ] mustard
- [ ] vegetable oil
- [ ] vinegar

WEEK 4
OTHER ITEMS

OTHER ITEMS

HEALTHY EATING HABITS
to Keep You on the Road to Success

EATING OUT: In your efforts to lose weight and get healthy, you can still eat out and enjoy yourself. It's all about making simple choices that will keep you on your ROUTE TO HEALTH.

- Order foods on the menu that are steamed, baked or broiled instead of fried.

- Avoid cream sauces and gravy and try to pick out items that are a healthy addition to your diet.

- Ask your server to bring a carryout box when he delivers your meal, then immediately put half of your meal into the box so you aren't tempted to eat it all.

- While you wait for your food, drink a full eight ounce glass of water. It's good for you and will fill you up a bit before your meal.

- Skip the dessert cart, but if you just can't pass up something sweet, order a sorbet or strawberries. If you do order dessert, get a few forks and share the treat with your friends.

- Portion control ALERT! Be careful at places with all-you-can-eat buffets. It's difficult to resist the temptation of overeating and making multiple trips.

CRAVINGS: This one simple word can get you off track on your ROUTE TO HEALTH. Do you practically hear the donuts, chocolate or pizza calling your name? Everything in moderation is good, so these cravings can be tamed by doing a few simple things.

- Try to use your "craving foods" as a reward after a week of eating healthy and exercise.

- When you are craving something like a chocolate bar, try breaking off a 1/4 of it and stick the rest in a bag in the freezer.

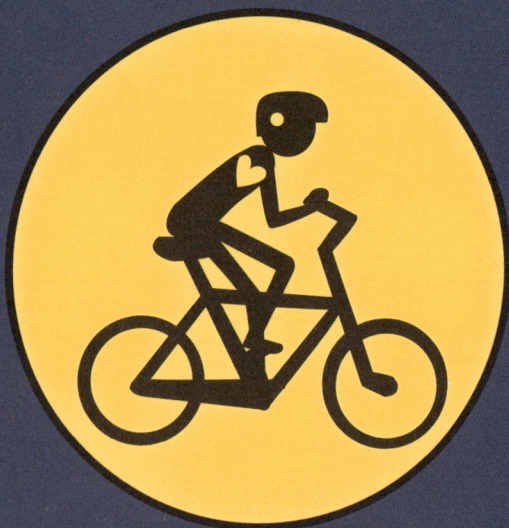

EXERCISE

Not only makes you healthy but makes you feel better!

Let's face it: exercise can be difficult to squeeze into your already busy schedule. But did you know that you don't have to run a marathon every day to get healthy? Exercise is a great way to relieve stress, brighten your mood, train your heart and make you feel like you're doing something great for yourself.

The health experts at www.MyPyramid.gov recommend at least 30 minutes of activity three to five days per week. However, 30 minutes a day is even better for you. If you don't have 30 minutes to do your exercises, then do 15 minutes in the morning and 15 minutes at night. Getting moving--whenever you can and however you can--is what counts.

If you are trying to prevent weight gain, most people need about 60 minutes of physical activity on most days. To keep off lost pounds, many people need 60-90 minutes of physical activity!

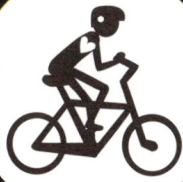

FAST FACTS
FOR YOUR
ROUTE TO HEALTH

Why in the world would I want to exercise? Of course the easy path is to sit on the couch and watch a movie, but getting your body moving has so many benefits. When physical activity is part of your daily life, it will change the way you feel overall and improve your self image.

DAILY EXERCISE HELPS...

- Control your weight

- Reduce your risk of heart disease

- Reduce your risk of type 2 diabetes

- Reduce your risk of some cancers

- Strengthen your bones and muscles

- Improve your balance and coordination

- Improve your mental health and mood

- Improve your ability to do daily activities

- Increase your chances of living longer

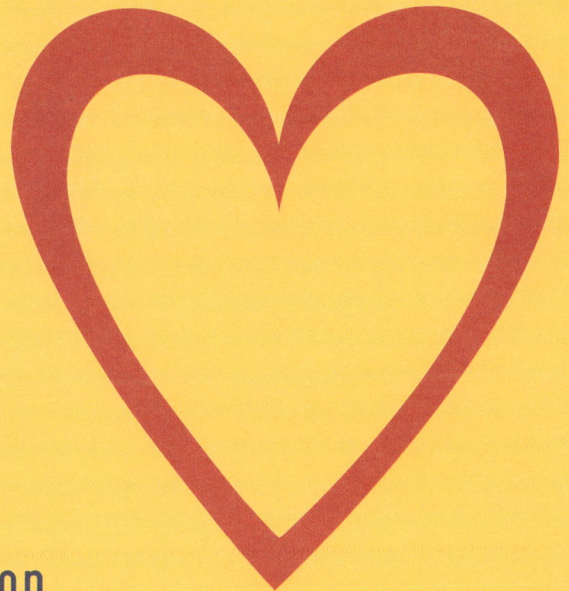

HOW TO GET YOUR BODY MOVING:

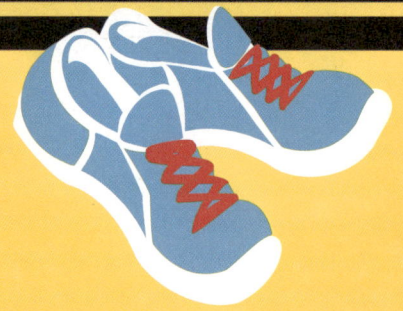

Everyone has a routine. We sleep, we eat, we work, take care of our children and our homes. All of that requires planning and scheduling time. Exercise is no different. Pick a specific time of day that works for you to get your body moving. If you aren't a morning person, DON'T try to convince yourself that you're getting up at 5 a.m. to work out before you go to work. Take your athletic shoes to work or school and enjoy a brisk walk around your building or in a nearby park during lunch time. If early evenings work better for you, stop by a local mall after work, put on your athletic shoes and walk in a place that is both safe and climate controlled. Do you have a friend that wants to become healthy too? Never underestimate the power of a workout buddy. He or she can keep you moving when you don't feel like it. A fun conversation on a long walk with a partner makes that workout time fly by. What about the health of your kids and pets? They all love to get outside. Walking with your kids allows you to spend quality time with them and get exercise at the same time. While you're walking with them, you could start a tradition by sharing the best thing that happened to you that day and what you're excited about for tomorrow. Every step you take is a step in the right direction for your health.

Q. WHY EXERCISE?

A. Because it works your most important muscle, your HEART, makes you feel better and releases endorphins!

AEROBIC EXERCISE: physical exercise that intends to improve the oxygen system.

GET YOUR BODY KICK-STARTED & EXERCISE!

1) Mow the lawn with a push mower. You'll get some fresh air and exercise.

2) Rent an exercise video from the library and get your body moving.

3) Do some housecleaning. Get some exercise and get organized at the same time!

4) Take the stairs in a building instead of the elevator to get your heart pumping!

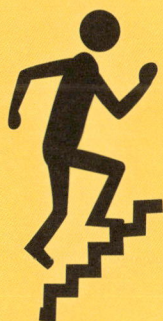

5) Get outside and go to the park and take a long walk.

6) Think about riding a bike to work and get in your daily exercise.

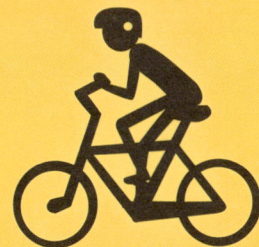

7) During your lunch hour, eat a light lunch and walk for the remaining time.

8) When going to a store, park your car at the furthest spot and get a brisk walk.

9) Join a recreational softball, baseball, soccer, tennis or basketball league.

10) Take your pet for a walk and get both of you heart healthy.

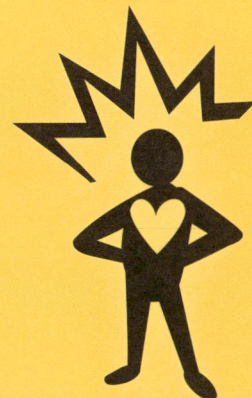

WEBSITES FOR MORE EXERCISE INFO:
www.startsmartforyourhealth.com
www.mypyramid.gov

EXERCISES for your ROUTE to HEALTH

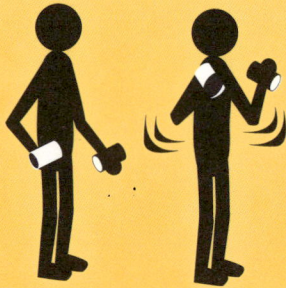

SOUP CAN CURLS

Put soup cans in each hand, elbows touching rib cage, palms facing up. Slowly curl your forearms up to your shoulders and back down. Repeat.

SEATED CHAIR BENDS

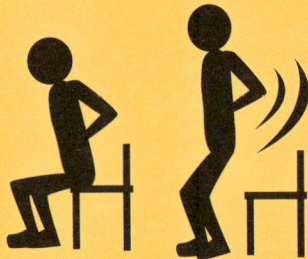

Put a chair up against a stationary wall. With your back to the chair, stand with feet 12" apart. Place your hands on your waist and sit down slowly, then stand up. Repeat.

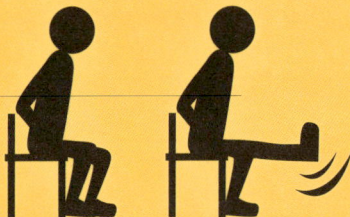

CHAIR LEG LIFTS

Sit in a chair with legs 6" apart. Slowly lift your leg until it is straight. Bend it back down. Alternate legs. Repeat.

WALL PUSH UPS

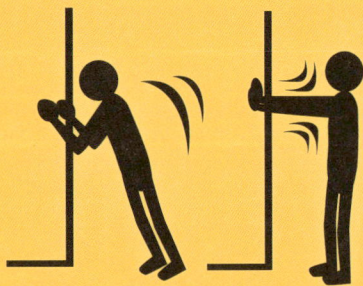

Stand arm length distance from a wall. Put your hands on the wall at shoulder height 12" apart. Slowly bend elbows and use your weight against your arms. Push your arms straight. Repeat.

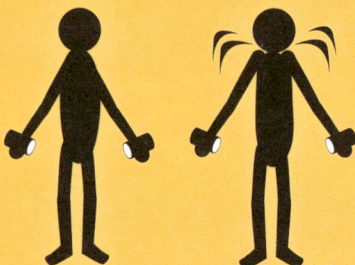

SOUP CAN SHOULDER SHRUGS

With soup cans in each hand, extend straight arms out 8-12" from your body. Move both shoulders up and down. Repeat.

GOALS

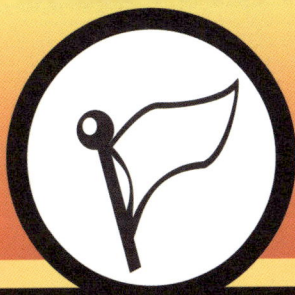

This section is designed to remind you of the goals you establish after you read the following sections in the book. Once you have read about nutrition, shopping, exercise and healthy habits, establishing your goals and then putting them into action will get you to the point of feeling healthier and living a more healthy life style. It's okay to leave this blank until you have read through each section. Take time to make real goals for each topic... because this route is all about you!

I want to feel more healthy about myself because _____

_____

I will achieve more health by doing _____

_____

I want to eat more healthy because _____

_____

I will make sure I eat healthy by doing _____

_____

It is important to me to stay active and exercise because _____

_____

I will stay on my exercise plan by doing _____

_____

MY 4 WEEK PLAN

MY DAILY HEALTHY EATING GOAL

_____

_____

_____

Color in the healthy eating circle on each day that you complete your goal

MY DAILY EXERCISE GOAL

_____

_____

_____

Every day you are active or exercise place an "x" in the day with a pen or pencil

MY DAILY HEALTHY HABIT

_____

_____

_____

Color in the Healthy Habits circle each day you complete your goal

Write the days/dates in the calendar from

SUNDAY	MONDAY	TU

SDAY	WEDNESDAY	THURSDAY	FRIDAY	SATURDAY

Some of the Reasons Why You May Want to Take a New ROUTE TO HEALTH

I WANT A STRONG BODY

I WANT TO BE MORE HEALTHY AND FEEL MORE HEALTHY

I WANT TO LIVE LONGER & FEEL BETTER

I WANT TO HAVE MORE ENERGY

I WANT TO BE ACTIVE WITH MY FAMILY

I WANT TO BE IN MORE CONTROL OF WHAT I EAT & HOW MUCH

I WANT TO BE ABLE TO ACHIEVE A GOAL I SET FOR MYSELF

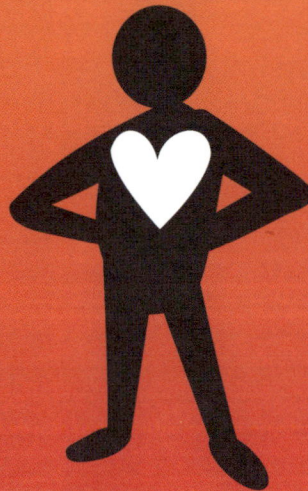

I WANT TO LOOK GREAT IN MY FAVORITE CLOTHES

I WANT TO SEE HEALTHY RESULTS FOR MYSELF

I WANT TO LIVE THE BEST HEALTHY LIFE I CAN

I WANT A MORE HEALTHY LIFESTYLE

I WANT TO LOSE WEIGHT

Flip this page out for a calendar!

I will stay on a **4** week plan for good habits because _____

_____

I will stay on my **4** week plan by doing _____

_____

I want to lose weight because _____

_____

I will stay focused on my weight loss by doing _____

_____

GET MOVIN' FOR YOUR HEART AND FOR YOU!

YOU CAN DO IT!

SHOW YOUR "HEALTHY STYLE" BY LIVING A BETTER LIFE!

CHOOSE YOUR HEALTH FOR THE ONES YOU LOVE!

A HEALTHIER LIFE IS AHEAD FOR YOU!

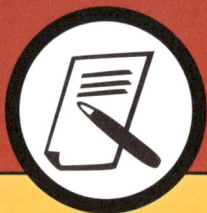

MY JOURNAL

Write a few sentences on how you are feeling about your new healthy changes and starting your ROUTE TO HEALTH.

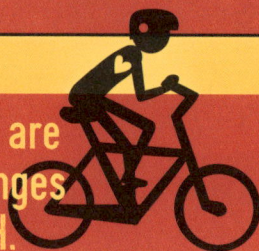

It's a great day to get started on YOUR ROUTE TO HEALTH!

_____
_____
_____
_____
_____

DAY 1

How do you feel today? (circle one)

How do you feel about your diet today? (circle one)

How do you feel about exercise today? (circle one)

What happened today that was great? _____

What happened today that was difficult? _____

If so, why was it difficult? _____

FOOD YOU ATE/CALORIES

| Breakfast | | | Dinner | | | TOTAL CALORIES | |
| Lunch | | | Snacks | | | | |

DAY 2

How do you feel today? (circle one)

How do you feel about your diet today? (circle one)

How do you feel about exercise today? (circle one)

What happened today that was great? _____

What happened today that was difficult? _____

If so, why was it difficult?

FOOD YOU ATE/CALORIES

| Breakfast | | | Dinner | | | TOTAL CALORIES | |
| Lunch | | | Snacks | | | | |

DAY 3

How do you feel today?
(circle one)

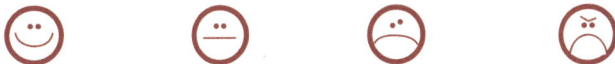

How do you feel about your diet today?
(circle one)

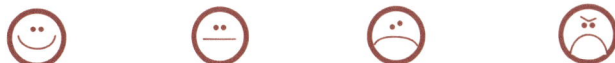

How do you feel about exercise today?
(circle one)

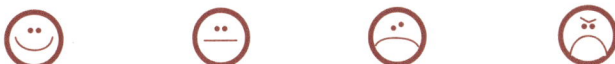

What happened today that was great? _____

What happened today that was difficult? _____

If so, why was it difficult? _____

FOOD YOU ATE/CALORIES

Breakfast			Dinner			TOTAL	
Lunch			Snacks			CALORIES	

DAY 4

How do you feel today?
(circle one)

How do you feel about your diet today?
(circle one)

How do you feel about exercise today?
(circle one)

What happened today that was great? _____

What happened today that was difficult? _____

If so, why was it difficult? _____

FOOD YOU ATE/CALORIES

Breakfast			Dinner			TOTAL	
Lunch			Snacks			CALORIES	

DAY 5

How do you feel today?
(circle one)

How do you feel about your diet today?
(circle one)

How do you feel about exercise today?
(circle one)

What happened today that was great? _____

What happened today that was difficult? _____

If so, why was it difficult? _____

FOOD YOU ATE/CALORIES

Breakfast			Dinner			TOTAL	
Lunch			Snacks			CALORIES	

DAY 6

How do you feel today?
(circle one)

How do you feel about your diet today?
(circle one)

How do you feel about exercise today?
(circle one)

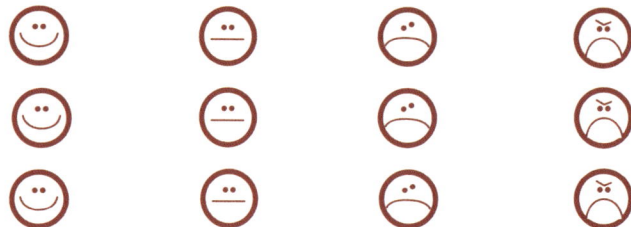

What happened today that was great? _____

What happened today that was difficult? _____

If so, why was it difficult? _____

FOOD YOU ATE/CALORIES

| Breakfast | | | Dinner | | | TOTAL | |
| Lunch | | | Snacks | | | CALORIES | |

DAY 7

How do you feel today?
(circle one)

How do you feel about your diet today?
(circle one)

How do you feel about exercise today?
(circle one)

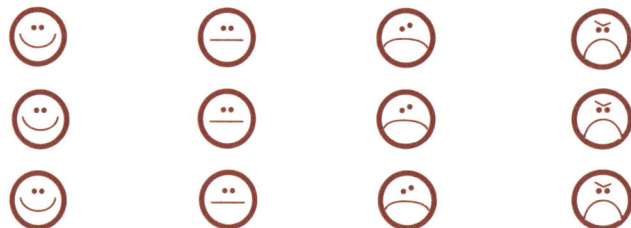

What happened today that was great? _____

What happened today that was difficult? _____

If so, why was it difficult? _____

FOOD YOU ATE/CALORIES

| Breakfast | | | Dinner | | | TOTAL | |
| Lunch | | | Snacks | | | CALORIES | |

DAY 8

How do you feel today?
(circle one)

How do you feel about your diet today?
(circle one)

How do you feel about exercise today?
(circle one)

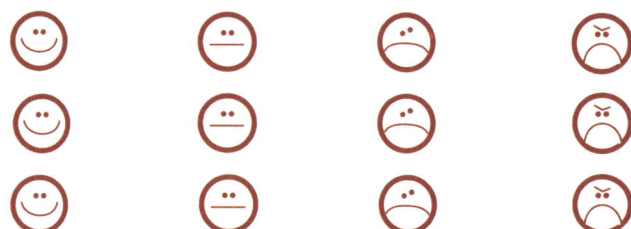

What happened today that was great? _____

What happened today that was difficult? _____

If so, why was it difficult? _____

FOOD YOU ATE/CALORIES

| Breakfast | | | Dinner | | | TOTAL | |
| Lunch | | | Snacks | | | CALORIES | |

DAY 9

How do you feel today?
(circle one)

How do you feel about your diet today?
(circle one)

How do you feel about exercise today?
(circle one)

What happened today that was great? _____

What happened today that was difficult? _____

If so, why was it difficult? _____

FOOD YOU ATE/CALORIES

Breakfast			Dinner			TOTAL	
Lunch			Snacks			CALORIES	

DAY 10

How do you feel today?
(circle one)

How do you feel about your diet today?
(circle one)

How do you feel about exercise today?
(circle one)

What happened today that was great? _____

What happened today that was difficult? _____

If so, why was it difficult? _____

FOOD YOU ATE/CALORIES

Breakfast			Dinner			TOTAL	
Lunch			Snacks			CALORIES	

DAY 11

How do you feel today?
(circle one)

How do you feel about your diet today?
(circle one)

How do you feel about exercise today?
(circle one)

What happened today that was great? _____

What happened today that was difficult? _____

If so, why was it difficult? _____

FOOD YOU ATE/CALORIES

Breakfast			Dinner			TOTAL	
Lunch			Snacks			CALORIES	

DAY 12

How do you feel today? (circle one)   😊 😐 🙁 😠

How do you feel about your diet today? (circle one)   😊 😐 🙁 😠

How do you feel about exercise today? (circle one)   😊 😐 🙁 😠

What happened today that was great? _____

What happened today that was difficult? _____

If so, why was it difficult? _____

FOOD YOU ATE/CALORIES

| Breakfast | / | Dinner | / | TOTAL | |
| Lunch | / | Snacks | / | CALORIES | |

DAY 13

How do you feel today? (circle one)   😊 😐 🙁 😠

How do you feel about your diet today? (circle one)   😊 😐 🙁 😠

How do you feel about exercise today? (circle one)   😊 😐 🙁 😠

What happened today that was great? _____

What happened today that was difficult? _____

If so, why was it difficult? _____

FOOD YOU ATE/CALORIES

| Breakfast | / | Dinner | / | TOTAL | |
| Lunch | / | Snacks | / | CALORIES | |

DAY 14

How do you feel today? (circle one)   😊 😐 🙁 😠

How do you feel about your diet today? (circle one)   😊 😐 🙁 😠

How do you feel about exercise today? (circle one)   😊 😐 🙁 😠

What happened today that was great? _____

What happened today that was difficult? _____

If so, why was it difficult? _____

FOOD YOU ATE/CALORIES

| Breakfast | / | Dinner | / | TOTAL | |
| Lunch | / | Snacks | / | CALORIES | |

DAY 15

How do you feel today? (circle one)

How do you feel about your diet today? (circle one)

How do you feel about exercise today? (circle one)

What happened today that was great? _____

What happened today that was difficult? _____

If so, why was it difficult? _____

FOOD YOU ATE/CALORIES

Breakfast			Dinner			TOTAL	
Lunch			Snacks			CALORIES	

DAY 16

How do you feel today? (circle one)

How do you feel about your diet today? (circle one)

How do you feel about exercise today? (circle one)

What happened today that was great? _____

What happened today that was difficult? _____

If so, why was it difficult? _____

FOOD YOU ATE/CALORIES

Breakfast			Dinner			TOTAL	
Lunch			Snacks			CALORIES	

DAY 17

How do you feel today? (circle one)

How do you feel about your diet today? (circle one)

How do you feel about exercise today? (circle one)

What happened today that was great? _____

What happened today that was difficult? _____

If so, why was it difficult? _____

FOOD YOU ATE/CALORIES

Breakfast			Dinner			TOTAL	
Lunch			Snacks			CALORIES	

DAY 18

How do you feel today?
(circle one)

How do you feel about your diet today?
(circle one)

How do you feel about exercise today?
(circle one)

What happened today that was great? _____

What happened today that was difficult? _____

If so, why was it difficult? _____

FOOD YOU ATE/CALORIES

Breakfast			Dinner			TOTAL	
Lunch			Snacks			CALORIES	

DAY 19

How do you feel today?
(circle one)

How do you feel about your diet today?
(circle one)

How do you feel about exercise today?
(circle one)

What happened today that was great? _____

What happened today that was difficult? _____

If so, why was it difficult? _____

FOOD YOU ATE/CALORIES

Breakfast			Dinner			TOTAL	
Lunch			Snacks			CALORIES	

DAY 20

How do you feel today?
(circle one)

How do you feel about your diet today?
(circle one)

How do you feel about exercise today?
(circle one)

What happened today that was great? _____

What happened today that was difficult? _____

If so, why was it difficult? _____

FOOD YOU ATE/CALORIES

Breakfast			Dinner			TOTAL	
Lunch			Snacks			CALORIES	

DAY 21

How do you feel today?
(circle one)

How do you feel about your diet today?
(circle one)

How do you feel about exercise today?
(circle one)

What happened today that was great? _____

What happened today that was difficult? _____

If so, why was it difficult? _____

FOOD YOU ATE/CALORIES

Breakfast		Dinner		TOTAL	
Lunch		Snacks		CALORIES	

DAY 22

How do you feel today?
(circle one)

How do you feel about your diet today?
(circle one)

How do you feel about exercise today?
(circle one)

What happened today that was great? _____

What happened today that was difficult? _____

If so, why was it difficult? _____

FOOD YOU ATE/CALORIES

Breakfast		Dinner		TOTAL	
Lunch		Snacks		CALORIES	

DAY 23

How do you feel today?
(circle one)

How do you feel about your diet today?
(circle one)

How do you feel about exercise today?
(circle one)

What happened today that was great? _____

What happened today that was difficult? _____

If so, why was it difficult? _____

FOOD YOU ATE/CALORIES

Breakfast		Dinner		TOTAL	
Lunch		Snacks		CALORIES	

DAY 24

How do you feel today?
(circle one)

How do you feel about your diet today?
(circle one)

How do you feel about exercise today?
(circle one)

What happened today that was great? _____

What happened today that was difficult? _____

If so, why was it difficult? _____

FOOD YOU ATE/CALORIES

| Breakfast | | | Dinner | | | TOTAL | |
| Lunch | | | Snacks | | | CALORIES | |

DAY 25

How do you feel today?
(circle one)

How do you feel about your diet today?
(circle one)

How do you feel about exercise today?
(circle one)

What happened today that was great? _____

What happened today that was difficult? _____

If so, why was it difficult? _____

FOOD YOU ATE/CALORIES

| Breakfast | | | Dinner | | | TOTAL | |
| Lunch | | | Snacks | | | CALORIES | |

DAY 26

How do you feel today?
(circle one)

How do you feel about your diet today?
(circle one)

How do you feel about exercise today?
(circle one)

What happened today that was great? _____

What happened today that was difficult? _____

If so, why was it difficult? _____

FOOD YOU ATE/CALORIES

| Breakfast | | | Dinner | | | TOTAL | |
| Lunch | | | Snacks | | | CALORIES | |

DAY 27

How do you feel today?
(circle one)

How do you feel about your diet today?
(circle one)

How do you feel about exercise today?
(circle one)

What happened today that was great? _____

What happened today that was difficult? _____

If so, why was it difficult? _____

FOOD YOU ATE/CALORIES

| Breakfast | | | Dinner | | | TOTAL | |
| Lunch | | | Snacks | | | CALORIES | |

DAY 28

How do you feel today?
(circle one)

How do you feel about your diet today?
(circle one)

How do you feel about exercise today?
(circle one)

What happened today that was great? _____

What happened today that was difficult? _____

If so, why was it difficult? _____

FOOD YOU ATE/CALORIES

| Breakfast | | | Dinner | | | TOTAL | |
| Lunch | | | Snacks | | | CALORIES | |

Write a few sentences on how you are feeling about your new healthy changes and starting your ROUTE TO HEALTH.

_____

_____

_____

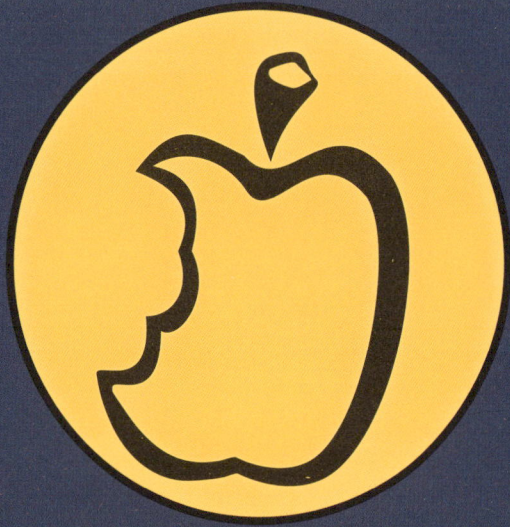

HEALTHY EATING...

TAKE A BITE OUT OF LIVING A BETTER LIFE FOR YOURSELF!

Let's face it, eating healthy isn't easy. With busy schedules it is hard to make the best choices for our bodies. The one thing your body does know is when it is getting a healthy and balanced diet. When you eat better, you feel better. Think of it like this... what if you filled your car's gas tank with water instead of gasoline? It wouldn't run quite right. Same with your body. When you don't give it the nutrition it needs, it doesn't run quite right either.

In this section we are going to look at healthy food choices that will help your body undertake its journey with as much energy as possible.

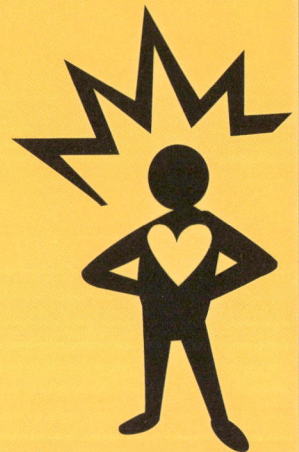

Q: WHY HEALTHY EATING?

A: Because it helps your overall health and gives you energy!

NUTRITION: The processes by which an animal or plant takes in and makes use of food substances.